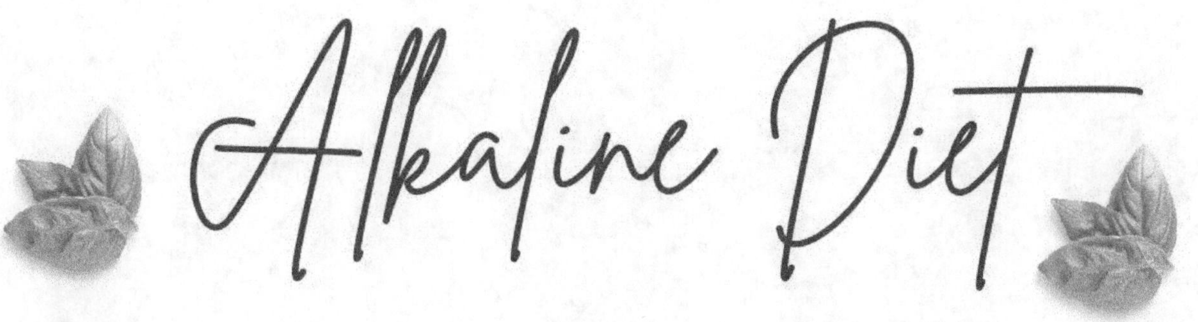

Alkaline Diet

Cancer Cookbook

For Beginners

Transforming Health, Fighting Inflammation, Preventing Cancer, and Savoring Culinary Delights

30-DAY Meal Plan | **100+** Recipes | **BONUS** Ebook | **5 WEEKS** Meal Plan Template

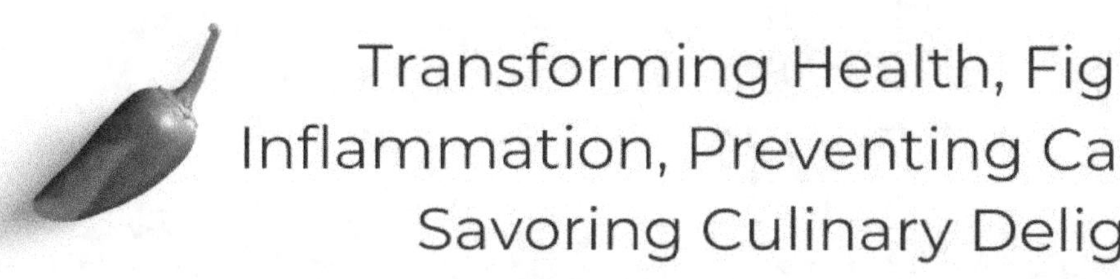

Sarah William

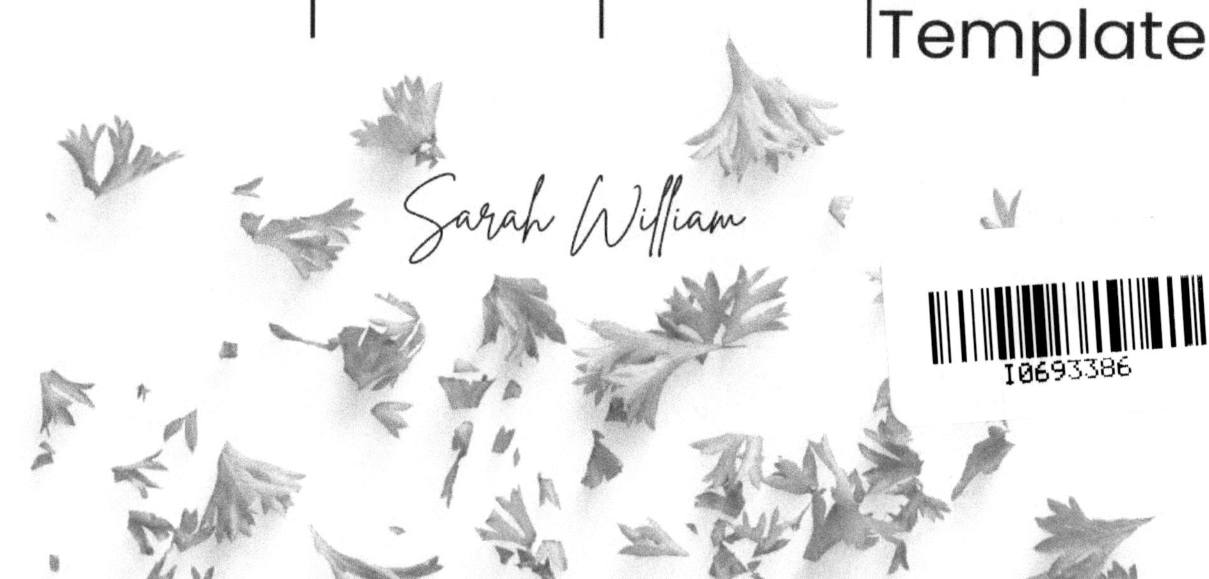

Table of Contents

Dedication

To all those who strive for a healthier tomorrow, May this book serve as a guiding light on your journey to wellness.

Introduction

This is the "Alkaline Diet Cancer Cookbook for Beginners." Welcome. We take a tour through the intriguing realm of the alkaline diet and its possible role in cancer prevention in this book.

Millions of people worldwide are impacted by the complicated illness known as cancer. Even though cancer therapy and management have advanced significantly, finding practical preventive measures is still a continuous challenge. Recent studies indicate that dietary decisions are critical in preventing cancer, with the alkaline diet gaining popularity due to its alleged health advantages.

The idea that the body's pH should be balanced is the foundation of the alkaline diet. It suggests that eating foods that support alkalinity will improve internal conditions and perhaps lessen oxidative stress and inflammation, two things linked to the onset and spread of cancer. The goal of the alkaline diet is to promote general health and well-being by focusing on entire, plant-based meals and reducing acidic foods.

We examine the foundations of the alkaline diet in this cookbook, including its tenets, advantages supported by research, and possible connections to cancer prevention. We want to provide you with useful tools and resources to include alkaline-rich foods in your regular meals, based on our study and scientific investigation.

We start by establishing the foundation for knowledge about pH balance and the differences between foods that are acidic and those that are alkaline. The complex link between nutrition and cancer is then explored, with an emphasis on how dietary habits might affect cancer risk and development. Our goal is to enable you to make knowledgeable decisions about your eating habits by providing you with a blend of scientific knowledge and practical examples.

The main focus of this cookbook is a selection of savory and filling dishes that are meant to make the switch to an alkaline diet easy and enjoyable. Every dish, which ranges from colorful breakfast bowls to filling main meals and decadent desserts, is carefully designed to highlight the variety of alkaline-forming items you have on hand.

We look at supplementary lifestyle practices outside of the kitchen that might help you on your path to perfect health. Our comprehensive counsel aims to nourish body, mind, and spirit, including everything from stress management strategies to mindful movement activities.

We invite you to approach the alkaline diet with an open mind, curiosity, and spirit of exploration as you set out on this gastronomic journey. Keep in mind that every meal is a chance to feed oneself from the inside out and that little adjustments may have a big impact.

This cookbook is your travel companion on the road to wellness, whether your goals are to lower your risk of cancer, assist a loved one in their recovery, or just adopt a better diet. I hope it encourages you to experience the life-changing potential of whole foods and set out on a path to bright health and vigor.

Understanding the Alkaline Diet

Examining the alkaline diet theoretically entails investigating its foundational ideas, putative modes of action, and prospective health consequences. Let's take a theoretical trip to get a deeper understanding of the alkaline diet:

pH Balance and Body Chemistry: The measurement of an alkaline or acidic solution, known as pH balance, is the foundation of the alkaline diet. The body's pH equilibrium is essential for many physiological functions, such as immunological response, cellular metabolism, and enzyme activity. Theoretically, proponents of an alkaline diet contend that eating foods high in alkalinity may support the body's normal pH levels, thereby supporting general health and well-being.

Alkaline-Forming Foods: The foundation of an alkaline diet is the consumption of foods that, after digestion, are thought to have a net alkalizing impact on the body. Fruits, vegetables, nuts, seeds, legumes, and certain whole grains are often included in this category of foods. Theoretically, those who adhere to an alkaline diet want to establish a more alkaline internal environment by emphasizing these nutrient-dense, plant-based foods, which supporters claim may have several health advantages.

Acidic Foods and pH Imbalance: On the other hand, it's thought that eating acidic foods, such as meat, dairy, refined sweets, and processed meals, will make your body more acidic. Theoretically, eating too many acidic foods may upset the pH balance and make the internal environment more acidic. This, according to some advocates of the alkaline diet, may lead to inflammation, oxidative stress, and a higher risk of developing chronic illnesses like cancer.

Possible Mechanisms of Action: The alkaline diet's supposed health advantages may be due to several processes. Alkaline-forming foods, for instance, are often high in vitamins, minerals, antioxidants, and phytonutrients—all of which have been shown to have anti-inflammatory and antioxidant qualities. Alkaline-forming foods also tend to be low in saturated fat and rich in fiber, which may help with weight management, cardiovascular health, and digestive health—all of which may affect the risk of cancer.

Cancer Prevention Theory: The alkaline diet may have some potential uses, including cancer prevention. Some argue that cancer cells may be less likely to proliferate in an environment that is kept slightly alkaline internally by eating a slightly alkaline diet. This theory is based on the idea that cancer cells can multiply more easily in an acidic environment and that increasing alkalinity may prevent cancer from spreading and growing. It's crucial to remember that this theory is still hypothetical and that there is little, conflicting scientific data to support an alkaline diet's ability to prevent cancer.

Unique Variability and Things to Take into Account: Theoretically, different people may react differently to the alkaline diet depending on things like genetics, lifestyle choices, general eating patterns, and pre-existing medical issues. Furthermore, there is no one-size-fits-all alkaline diet; what works for one person may not work for another. People must proceed cautiously when making dietary modifications and seek advice from medical specialists or trained dietitians before making substantial dietary adjustments.

In conclusion, studying the theoretical underpinnings, plausible mechanisms of action, and prospective health implications—including its possible involvement in cancer prevention—is necessary to comprehend the alkaline diet. The concepts of the alkaline diet provide insights into the relationship between pH balance, general well-being, and food, even if it is still a subject of discussion and current study.

Exploring the Link Between Diet and Cancer Prevention

There is a lot of scientific interest and research on the relationship between nutrition and cancer prevention. Notwithstanding the nuanced and intricate nature of the link, evidence indicates that dietary decisions have a major impact on cancer risk. Now let's explore this relationship:

Nutrient Density and Antioxidants: Vital vitamins, minerals, fiber, and antioxidants may be obtained from a diet high in nutrient-dense foods such as fruits, vegetables, whole grains, nuts, seeds, and legumes. Antioxidants aid in the body's defense against dangerous free radicals, which may cause cell damage and accelerate the onset of cancer. Eating a variety of vibrant plant foods guarantees a wide range of antioxidants, which may lower the risk of cancer.

Anti-inflammatory Properties: In their genesis and progression, several cancer types have been linked to chronic inflammation. The Mediterranean diet and plant-based diets, for example, are linked to reduced levels of inflammation because they place a strong focus on whole, minimally processed foods, healthy fats (such as omega-3 fatty acids), and phytonutrients that have anti-inflammatory qualities. These diets may help lower the risk of cancer by reducing inflammation.

Weight control: Excessive body weight and obesity are known risk factors for several cancers, including pancreatic, colorectal, prostate, and breast cancers. The risk of obesity-related malignancies may be decreased by maintaining a healthy weight or, if required, facilitating weight reduction with a balanced diet that prioritizes whole foods and portion management.

Gut Microbiota and Fiber: A new study indicates that the trillions of bacteria and other microorganisms that live in the gastrointestinal system, known as the gut microbiota, are important players in immune response, inflammation, and metabolic regulation. Plant-based diets are high in dietary fiber, which acts as a prebiotic to support healthy gut flora. A varied and high-fiber diet promotes a healthy gut microbiota, which may lower the risk of cancer via several processes, such as improved immunological surveillance and inflammatory regulation.

Dietary Decisions and Carcinogen Exposure: Certain dietary decisions may have a direct impact on one's exposure to carcinogens, chemicals that promote cancer development, as well as other dangerous compounds. For instance, eating a lot of processed meats and meats that have been grilled or charred exposes people to chemicals that may cause cancer, like polycyclic aromatic hydrocarbons and heterocyclic amines. On the other hand, consuming less processed and red meat and opting for lean protein sources, along with better cooking techniques, might help reduce your exposure to these carcinogens.

Alcohol and cancer chance: Drinking alcohol has been linked to a higher chance of developing breast, liver, colorectal, and esophageal cancers, among other cancers. Reducing alcohol use or giving it up completely may help lower the risk of cancer, especially when paired with other healthy lifestyle choices like quitting smoking, eating a balanced diet, and getting regular exercise.

The connection between diet and cancer prevention emphasizes how crucial it is to follow a varied, balanced diet high in plant-based foods and to limit intake of processed and possibly cancer-causing foods. Through educated food selection and the prioritization of whole, nutrient-dense meals, people may be able to lower their risk of cancer and improve their general health and well-being. Our understanding of the complex relationship between nutrition and cancer is still being deepened by ongoing research, which informs both individual lifestyle modifications and public health recommendations.

Chapter 1

Foundations of the Alkaline Diet

The alkaline diet is founded on the concept of the body's pH equilibrium. Here is a description of the fundamental ideas behind the alkaline diet:

Balance: The pH scale, which goes from 0 to 14, with 7 being neutral, determines how acidic or alkaline a thing is. The human body maintains ideal physiological function by controlling its pH levels within a certain range. The alkaline diet's proponents believe that eating certain foods may affect the body's pH balance, to keep it slightly alkaline—pH 7.35 to 7.45, on average.

Foods that are alkaline vs. acidic: The alkaline diet groups foods according to how they may impact the pH levels of the body. After digestion, meals that produce an alkaline residue leave an acidic residue behind, whereas those that produce an acidic residue leave an alkaline residue. Fruits, vegetables, nuts, seeds, legumes, and certain whole grains are examples of foods that produce an alkaline environment; meat, dairy, eggs, refined grains, processed meals, and some sweets are examples of foods that form an acidic environment.

Health Benefits: Advocates of the alkaline diet assert that keeping the body's pH slightly alkaline can have several positive effects on health, including better digestion, more energy, stronger immunity, less inflammation, and a decreased risk of chronic illnesses like cancer, heart disease, and osteoporosis. This is because, compared to an acidic environment, an alkaline environment is thought to be less favorable for the onset and spread of illness.

Nutrient Density: A fundamental feature of the alkaline diet is its focus on complete, nutrient-dense foods. Foods that generate an alkaline environment are often high in vitamins, minerals, antioxidants, and phytonutrients—all of which are critical for good health and well-being overall. Those who follow an alkaline diet prioritize these items to maximize their intake of nutrients and promote optimum physiological performance.

Hydration: The importance of staying hydrated is a fundamental tenet of the alkaline diet. Advocates advise drinking alkaline-forming liquids, including water with lime or lemon, to keep the body hydrated and alkaline. Maintaining cellular function, detoxification procedures, and general wellness all depend on getting enough water.

Limitations and Considerations: Although the alkaline diet encourages the eating of plant-based, high-nutrient foods, there are some restrictions and things to keep in mind. Critics argue that dietary changes are unlikely to significantly affect blood pH levels because the body has strong systems for controlling pH equilibrium. Furthermore, certain alkaline diets may exclude nutrient-dense foods like lean proteins and entire grains, which, if improperly balanced, may result in nutritional deficits.

The idea of pH balance and the impact of food decisions on the body's internal environment form the basis of the alkaline diet. Alkaline-forming foods and nutritional density are prioritized by proponents to promote general health and well-being. But it's crucial to approach the alkaline diet with balance and critical thought, taking into account food choices and individual demands.

Principles of pH Balance in the Body

Grasp the alkaline diet and its alleged health advantages requires a grasp of the fundamentals of pH equilibrium in the body. The following is a discussion of pH balancing principles:

The term pH relates to the "potential of hydrogen" and is used to assess how acidic or alkaline a solution is. The pH scale has a neutral pH of 7 and a range of 0 to 14. A pH of less than 7 denotes acidity, whereas a pH of more than 7 denotes alkalinity. The body sustains diverse pH values in distinct bodily compartments and fluids to facilitate vital physiological processes.

Blood pH Control: The pH level in the blood is one of the most strictly controlled in the body. The pH of arterial blood is normally kept within a small range of 7.35 to 7.45; any deviation from this range causes the body to react physiologically to return the blood to equilibrium. To maintain blood pH homeostasis, the body uses a variety of buffering systems, such as the blood's bicarbonate buffer and respiratory and renal processes.

The importance of pH equilibrium cannot be overstated. Both general health and good cellular function depend on it. The body's metabolic processes depend on enzymes, which have ideal pH ranges within which they may operate. A pH outside of the ideal range may damage biological functions and reduce the activity of enzymes. Sustaining the integrity of cell membranes and controlling ion transport across them both depend on maintaining the right pH equilibrium.

Base-Acid Balance: Acids are produced by the body as waste products of metabolic activities such as cellular respiration and nutritional degradation. It is necessary to neutralize or remove these acids to avoid pH changes that might be harmful to health. Proteins and bicarbonate ions are examples of buffers that support pH equilibrium by neutralizing acids. Through adjustments to the blood's levels of bicarbonate ions and carbon dioxide, the kidneys and lungs play important roles in maintaining acid-base balance.

<u>Dietary Impact on pH Balance:</u> Although the body closely controls blood pH, proponents of the alkaline diet contend that other bodily fluids and tissues may have their pH levels affected by food choices. They suggest that eating foods high in alkalinity may raise the alkalinity of the internal environment, which may have positive effects on immunity, detoxification, and inflammation reduction. Nevertheless, there is little scientific proof to back up these assertions, and the body's capacity to maintain pH balance is intricate and multifaceted.

<u>Potential Health Repercussions:</u> According to some studies, long-term pH imbalance aberrations may be linked to specific medical disorders such as metabolic acidosis or alkalosis. Still up for debate, however, are the importance of these variations and how they affect general health. While eating more alkaline-forming foods is encouraged by the alkaline diet to boost health, it's important to approach dietary changes cautiously and take individual requirements and tastes into account.

Understanding pH balance is essential to comprehending the alkaline diet and its alleged health benefits. Although the blood pH is tightly regulated by the body, there is continuous discussion and study about the impact of food choices on other bodily fluids and tissues. Maintaining general health and well-being requires a balanced diet and way of living.

Alkaline vs. Acidic Foods: What to Eat and What to Avoid

The foundation of the alkaline diet is an understanding of the differences between foods that are acidic and those that are alkaline. Let's talk about the types of foods that are acidic and alkaline, as well as what you should and shouldn't eat:

Foods that leave an alkaline residue after digestion are known as alkaline-forming foods, and they may help to create a more alkaline internal environment in the body.

<u>Foods that generate an alkaline environment include:</u>

- ✓ Fruits include melons, avocados, citrus fruits, bananas, apples, and berries.
- ✓ Vegetables: These include root vegetables (carrots, beets, and sweet potatoes), cruciferous vegetables (broccoli, cauliflower, and Brussels sprouts), and other veggies like cucumber and bell peppers.
- ✓ Nuts and Seeds: hemp, flax, chia, walnut, and almond seeds.
- ✓ Legumes include peas, beans, chickpeas, and lentils.
- ✓ Whole grains: amaranth, buckwheat, millet, and quinoa.

These foods are generally high in vitamins, minerals, fiber, and other nutrients and are recommended for their potential health benefits.

Foods That Form Acids:

- ✓ Meals that leave an acidic residue after digestion are known as acidic-forming meals because they may help create an internally acidic environment in the body.
- ✓ Foods that might cause acid reflux include:
- ✓ Meat (particularly red meat), chicken, fish, eggs, and dairy products (milk, cheese, and yogurt) are examples of animal proteins.
- ✓ Processed foods include packaged snacks, processed meats, refined grains, and sugary snacks.
- ✓ Refined sugars include high-fructose corn syrup, white sugar, and sugar-filled drinks.
- ✓ Fats: Fried meals, processed snacks, and baked products contain saturated and trans fats.
- ✓ A Few Grains are refined grains, including those found in pasta, white rice, and bread.

These foods are often deficient in nutrients and may pose health hazards, including oxidative stress, inflammation, and a higher chance of developing chronic illnesses.

Recommendations:

Consume More Foods That Form Alkaline: Try to eat a range of foods that create an alkaline diet, such as whole grains, fruits, vegetables, legumes, nuts, and seeds. These meals promote general health and well-being by offering vital nutrients.

Eat Less Acid-Forming Foods: While avoiding all items that cause acidity is not necessary, it is wise to consume less highly processed food, sweet snacks, refined grains, and animal protein. Instead, prioritize complete, high-nutrient meals that promote alkalinity and reinforce a well-rounded diet.

Pay Attention to Balance: Having a balanced diet is essential. Rather than obsessing about whether a meal is acidic or alkaline, concentrate on eating a variety of whole foods, placing a strong emphasis on plant-based alternatives, and reducing processed and unhealthy foods.

Think About Individual Needs: When choosing a diet, it's important to take into account each person's unique dietary preferences, health objectives, and any underlying medical concerns. A licensed dietician or other healthcare expert may provide you with individualized advice based on your particular requirements.

Making dietary decisions and promoting general health and well-being may be made easier by knowing the difference between alkaline and acidic foods. People may be able to encourage a more balanced internal environment and lower their chance of developing chronic illnesses by prioritizing meals that generate an alkaline environment and reducing those that form an acidic one.

Benefits of an Alkaline-Forming Diet

Eating foods that, after digestion, leave an alkaline residue indicates that one is following an alkaline-forming diet, which may help to create a more alkaline internal environment in the body. Let's examine the possible advantages of adhering to an alkaline-forming diet:

Better Acid-Base Balance: Advocates of the alkaline diet contend that eating foods that are alkaline-forming may aid in keeping the body's pH level slightly alkaline, which is thought to be beneficial for optimum health. Blood pH is strictly regulated by the body, but advocates claim that increasing alkalinity in other bodily fluids and tissues may have advantages, including lowered inflammation, strengthened detoxification, and boosted immune system performance.

Increased Nutrient Intake: Foods that generate an alkaline environment are often high in nutrients, including vitamins, minerals, antioxidants, and phytonutrients. Alkaline diet mainstays such as fruits, vegetables, nuts, seeds, legumes, and whole grains are rich in vital elements that promote general health and well-being. People may maximize their nutritional intake and support good physiological function by making certain foods a priority.

Anti-inflammatory Effects: Because they are high in antioxidants and phytonutrients, many foods that generate an alkaline environment have an anti-inflammatory effect. Numerous chronic illnesses, including cancer, diabetes, and cardiovascular disease, are linked to chronic inflammation in its early stages. An alkaline-forming diet may help lower the risk of several conditions and improve general health by reducing inflammation.

Bone Health Encouragement: According to some studies, an alkaline-forming diet may be beneficial for bone health. Proponents of the alkaline diet contend that eating foods that are high in alkalinity will help lower the incidence of osteoporosis and bone fractures by encouraging a more alkaline environment inside the body, even if the research is not definitive. To properly comprehend the connection between dietary acid load and bone health, further study is necessary.

Weight management: foods that generate an alkaline environment are often high in fiber and low in calories, which may help with satiety and weight control. Additionally, those on an alkaline-forming diet may find it simpler to maintain a healthy weight or reach their weight reduction goals by emphasizing whole, minimally processed foods and minimizing intake of highly processed and calorie-dense foods.

Possible Cancer Prevention: Some studies indicate that an alkaline-forming diet may have consequences for cancer prevention, although the data is currently preliminary. Fruits, vegetables, and legumes are examples of foods that generate an alkaline environment and are high in antioxidants and phytochemicals, which have been shown to have anti-cancer effects. Furthermore, encouraging an alkaline internal environment may, in theory, make it harder for cancer cells to proliferate; however, further study is required in this area.

An alkaline-forming diet has many advantages, such as better acid-base balance, more nutrient-dense food intake, anti-inflammatory effects, potential support for bone health, benefits for weight management, and possible implications for cancer prevention. Giving priority to foods that create an alkaline environment may be an important part of a balanced and health-promoting diet, even if more research is required to fully understand the impact of the alkaline diet on health outcomes.

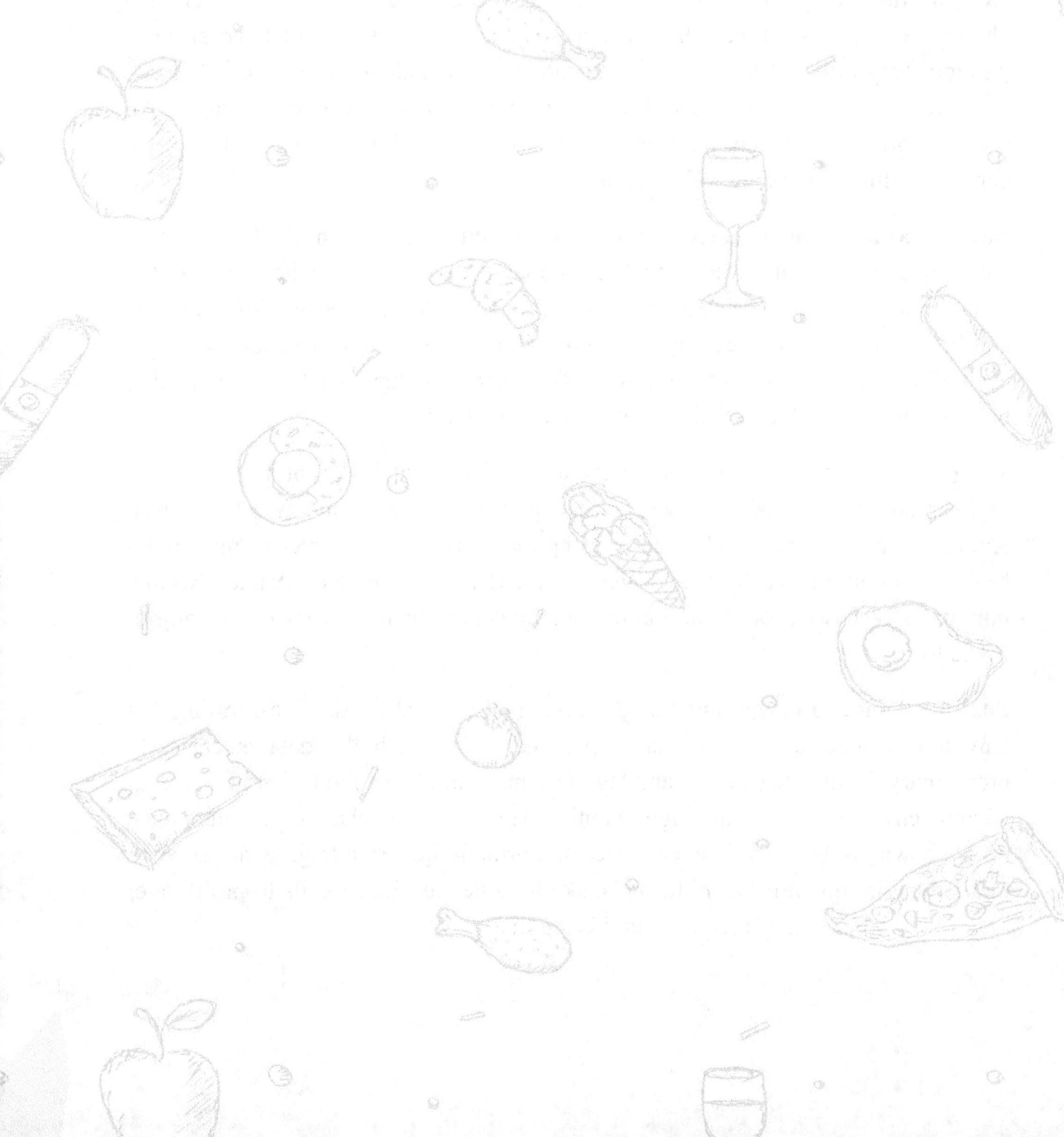

Chapter 2

Cancer Prevention and the Alkaline Diet

Eating foods that, after digestion, leave an alkaline residue indicates that one is following an alkaline-forming diet, which may help to create a more alkaline internal environment in the body. Let's examine the possible advantages of adhering to an alkaline-forming diet:

Better Acid-Base Balance: Advocates of the alkaline diet contend that eating foods that are alkaline-forming may aid in keeping the body's pH level slightly alkaline, which is thought to be beneficial for optimum health. Blood pH is strictly regulated by the body, but advocates claim that increasing alkalinity in other bodily fluids and tissues may have advantages, including lowered inflammation, strengthened detoxification, and boosted immune system performance.

Increased Nutrient Intake: Foods that generate an alkaline environment are often high in nutrients, including vitamins, minerals, antioxidants, and phytonutrients.

Alkaline diet mainstays such as fruits, vegetables, nuts, seeds, legumes, and whole grains are rich in vital elements that promote general health and well-being. People may maximize their nutritional intake and support good physiological function by making certain foods a priority.

Anti-inflammatory Effects: Because they are high in antioxidants and phytonutrients, many foods that generate an alkaline environment have an anti-inflammatory effect. Numerous chronic illnesses, including cancer, diabetes, and cardiovascular disease, are linked to chronic inflammation in its early stages. An alkaline-forming diet may help lower the risk of several conditions and improve general health by reducing inflammation.

Bone Health Encouragement: According to some studies, an alkaline-forming diet may be beneficial for bone health. Proponents of the alkaline diet contend that eating foods that are high in alkalinity will help lower the incidence of osteoporosis and bone fractures by encouraging a more alkaline environment inside the body, even if the research is not definitive. To properly comprehend the connection between dietary acid load and bone health, further study is necessary.

Weight management: foods that generate an alkaline environment are often high in fiber and low in calories, which may help with satiety and weight control. Additionally, those on an alkaline-forming diet may find it simpler to maintain a healthy weight or reach their weight reduction goals by emphasizing whole, minimally processed foods and minimizing intake of highly processed and calorie-dense foods.

Possible Cancer Prevention: Some studies indicate that an alkaline-forming diet may have consequences for cancer prevention, although the data is currently preliminary. Fruits, vegetables, and legumes are examples of foods that generate an alkaline environment and are high in antioxidants and phytochemicals, which have been shown to have anti-cancer effects. Furthermore, encouraging an alkaline internal environment may, in theory, make it harder for cancer cells to proliferate; however, further study is required in this area.

An alkaline-forming diet has many advantages, such as better acid-base balance, more nutrient-dense food intake, anti-inflammatory effects, potential support for bone health, benefits for weight management, and possible implications for cancer prevention. Giving priority to foods that create an alkaline environment may be an important part of a balanced and health-promoting diet, even if more research is required to fully understand the impact of the alkaline diet on health outcomes.

Exploring the Relationship Between Diet and Cancer

There is discussion and interest in the connection between cancer prevention and an alkaline diet. Although proponents of the alkaline diet contend that eating decisions that preserve an alkaline internal environment may lower the risk of cancer, there is little and conflicting scientific data to support this assertion. Let's investigate the potential connection between an alkaline diet and preventing cancer:

Possible Processes: *The alkaline diet may potentially prevent cancer via several mechanisms, including:*

Decreased Inflammation: Foods that generate an alkaline environment are generally high in phytonutrients and antioxidants, both of which have anti-inflammatory qualities. Eating an anti-inflammatory diet may potentially help reduce the risk of cancer since chronic inflammation has been linked to an elevated risk of the disease.

Enhanced immunological function: vitamins, minerals, and phytochemicals are among the nutrients that are included in alkaline-forming meals and are crucial for maintaining immunological function. Being able to recognize and eradicate malignant cells before they have the chance to spread requires a strong immune system.

Modified Tumor Microenvironment: Advocates of this theory argue that encouraging an alkaline internal environment may make the environment less conducive to cancer cell growth. There is a possibility that foods that generate an alkaline environment might prevent the development and spread of cancer, as cancer cells prefer to multiply in an acidic environment.

Goodness Against Cancer in Alkaline-Forming Foods: Fruits, vegetables, nuts, seeds, legumes, and other alkaline-forming foods are high in antioxidants, vitamins, minerals, and phytochemicals that have been shown to have anti-cancer effects. Broccoli and kale, for instance, are examples of cruciferous vegetables that contain chemicals that may help prevent certain forms of cancer.

Dietary Patterns and Cancer Risk: Observational research has shown links between an alkaline diet-like dietary pattern and a lower risk of developing certain malignancies. For instance, a decreased risk of colon cancer and other cancers has been linked to diets high in fruits, vegetables, whole grains, and legumes.

There is a need for more research: Although these postulated pathways and correlations are fascinating, it's important to understand that there is a lack of conflicting scientific data to establish a direct linkage between an alkaline diet and cancer prevention. More research is required to fully understand the potential advantages and limitations of the alkaline diet in this context, as there are currently insufficient controlled clinical studies, particularly evaluating its impact on cancer prevention.

An Equitable Strategy for Cancer Prevention: Healthy eating is just one aspect of cancer prevention's complex puzzle. A complete strategy for cancer prevention should also include other critical components, including keeping a healthy weight, engaging in regular physical exercise, abstaining from tobacco, consuming alcohol in moderation, and receiving frequent tests.

Although the alkaline diet has fascinating prospects for cancer prevention, further research is needed to determine if it lowers cancer risk. Adopting a balanced and evidence-based approach to cancer prevention is crucial, just like any other nutritional strategy. It should take into consideration individual requirements, preferences, and lifestyle variables. Speaking with a registered dietician or other healthcare expert may help you get individualized advice based on your unique health objectives and concerns.

Anti-inflammatory Effects of Alkaline Foods

The body uses inflammation as a normal immunological response to fend off infections and heal injured tissues. Chronic inflammation, however, has been linked to the onset and advancement of several chronic illnesses, including autoimmune disorders, diabetes, cancer, and cardiovascular disease. Studies indicate that the inflammatory response may be influenced by dietary choices, with certain foods having anti-inflammatory qualities. This conversation is about investigating the possible health benefits of alkaline diets and their anti-inflammatory properties.

Understanding Inflammation: Activating immune cells, releasing inflammatory mediators, and attracting immune cells to areas of damage or infection are all parts of the intricate biological process that is inflammation.

When the inflammatory response lasts for an extended period, it may cause tissue damage, poor healing, and immunological dysregulation. This is known as chronic inflammation.

Chronic inflammation may be caused by several lifestyle variables, including nutrition, stress, physical inactivity, and exposure to the environment.

Alkaline foods are those that leave an alkaline residue after digestion and may help to create a more alkaline internal environment in the body.

The alkaline diet's proponents believe that maintaining a slightly alkaline pH equilibrium may reduce inflammation and improve general health.

Although the blood pH is strictly regulated by the body, research is still being done on how food choices affect other bodily fluids and tissues.

Vitamin Density and Anti-Inflammatory Compounds: Nutrient-dense and abundant in vitamins, minerals, antioxidants, and phytochemicals, alkaline foods include fruits, vegetables, nuts, seeds, and legumes.

By modifying inflammatory pathways, lowering oxidative stress, and preventing the synthesis of pro-inflammatory mediators, some of these foods and substances have been shown to have anti-inflammatory qualities.

Particular Anti-Inflammatory Diets:

Leafy Greens: Rich in antioxidants like flavonoids and carotenoids, which have strong anti-inflammatory properties, spinach, kale, Swiss chard, and other leafy greens are also high in vitamins A, C, and K.

Nuts and Seeds: Almonds, walnuts, chia seeds, flaxseeds, and hemp seeds are excellent sources of omega-3 fatty acids, which have anti-inflammatory properties. Berries: Blueberries, strawberries, raspberries, and other berries are packed with antioxidants, particularly anthocyanins, which have been shown to reduce inflammation and oxidative stress.

Turmeric and ginger: These spices have been used for centuries in traditional medicine because they contain bioactive chemicals called curcumin and gingerol, which have strong anti-inflammatory properties.

Consequences for Health:

Eating a diet high in alkaline foods may help to reduce long-term inflammation and the chance of developing inflammation-related disorders.

People who consume a diet high in alkaline foods may find that their symptoms of chronic inflammatory diseases, including arthritis, inflammatory bowel disease, and cardiovascular disease, improve.

Adopting a balanced diet that consists of a range of nutrient-dense foods is crucial, as is taking into account other lifestyle variables that raise the risk of inflammation.

Because they are high in nutrients and contain bioactive chemicals that alter inflammatory pathways, alkaline foods have anti-inflammatory qualities. Increasing the amount of alkaline foods in the diet may help minimize long-term inflammation and reduce the risk of developing inflammation-related disorders. Individuals may enhance their general health and well-being by prioritizing complete, nutrient-dense meals in their diet choices.

Plant-Based Nutrition and Cancer Prevention

In recent years, there has been a significant increase in interest in plant-based diets due to their potential health benefits, including cancer prevention. Plant-based diets, which are high in fiber, phytochemicals, antioxidants, and other vital nutrients, have many health-promoting benefits that may help lower the chance of developing cancer. This talk examines the connection between cancer prevention and plant-based nutrition, emphasizing the main processes and data in favor of this dietary strategy.

Plant-based diets emphasize complete, minimally processed foods that come from plants, such as fruits, vegetables, whole grains, legumes, nuts, seeds, and plant-based sources of protein. These foods have a high nutrient density.

Naturally rich in vitamins, minerals, antioxidants, and phytochemicals, these foods are essential for immune system support, DNA repair, detoxification, and cellular health.

Eating a wide variety of plant-based meals guarantees a comprehensive range of nutrients that collaborate to support optimum health and might perhaps lower the chance of developing cancer.

Properties that are antioxidant and anti-inflammatory:

Fruits, vegetables, and other plant-based meals rich in antioxidants may help lower the body's oxidative stress by scavenging dangerous free radicals.

Several plant-based foods include anti-inflammatory qualities that may help reduce inflammation and its detrimental effects on cellular health. Chronic inflammation is a significant factor in cancer development.

It has been shown that phytochemicals from plant-based diets, such as flavonoids, carotenoids, and polyphenols, may alter inflammatory pathways and stop the development and spread of cancer cells.

Digestive Health and Fiber:

Dietary fiber, which is abundant in plant-based diets, is essential for promoting digestive health and preserving bowel regularity.

A sufficient amount of fiber has been linked to a lower risk of colorectal cancer, presumably because it helps to encourage the excretion of carcinogens, control gut bacteria, and lessen colon inflammation.

Plant-based diets are inherently low in cholesterol and saturated fat, but they do include good fats like monounsaturated and polyunsaturated fats, which may be found in nuts, seeds, avocados, and olive oil. They also contain omega-3 fatty acids.

Rich in fatty fish, flaxseeds, chia seeds, and walnuts, omega-3 fatty acids have anti-inflammatory qualities and may lower the incidence of breast and prostate cancer, among other malignancies.

Evidence in Favor of Plant-Based Dietary Interventions to Prevent Cancer:

Following a plant-based diet has been linked to a decreased risk of acquiring many cancers, including colon, breast, prostate, lung, and stomach cancer, according to several epidemiological studies.

Clinical trials and experimental investigations have provided mechanistic insights into the anti-cancer properties of plant-based meals, demonstrating that these foods can limit tumor development, induce apoptosis (cell death), and decrease cancer cell proliferation.

Realistic Suggestions:

To optimize the amount of nutrients and antioxidants in your diet, include a range of vibrant fruits and vegetables in your meals and snacks.

To increase fiber and nutritional content, choose whole grains like brown rice, quinoa, oats, and whole wheat instead of processed grains.

To enhance muscle health and encourage satiety, include plant-based protein sources like edamame, beans, lentils, tofu, and tempeh in your meals.

To improve taste and nutritional absorption, use healthy fats like olive oil, avocado, nuts, and seeds in cooking and meal preparation.

A diet high in plant-based nutrients has several health advantages, one of which may be its ability to prevent cancer. By placing a strong emphasis on whole, minimally processed plant-based foods, people may use plant-based nutrition to lower their risk of cancer and improve their general health and well-being. It is advantageous for both personal and planetary health to adopt a plant-based diet since it is good for the environment, animal welfare, and human health.

Chapter 3

Alkaline Diet and Cancer Cookbook

Breakfast Recipes for a Cancer-Preventive Diet

Green Smoothie Bowl

Prep Time: 5 minutes   Cook Time: 0 minute   Serving Size: 1 bowl

INGREDIENTS

1. 1 cup spinach
2. 1/2 cup kale
3. 1 ripe banana
4. 1/2 cup frozen berries (such as strawberries, blueberries, or raspberries)
5. 1/2 cup almond milk or coconut water
6. 1 tablespoon chia seeds
7. Optional toppings: sliced fruit, nuts, seeds, granola

PREPARATION

1. Blend spinach, kale, banana, berries, and almond milk or coconut water until smooth.
2. Pour the smoothie into a bowl.
3. Sprinkle chia seeds and add optional toppings as desired.

Quinoa Breakfast Bowl

Prep Time: 5 minutes Cook Time: 15 minutes (for quinoa) Serving Size: 1 bowl

INGREDIENTS

1. 1/2 cup cooked quinoa
2. 1/2 cup mixed berries
3. 1/4 cup sliced almonds
4. 1 tablespoon hemp seeds
5. 1 tablespoon maple syrup or honey (optional)
6. Dash of cinnamon

PREPARATION

1. Cook quinoa according to package instructions and let cool slightly.
2. In a bowl, combine cooked quinoa, mixed berries, sliced almonds, and hemp seeds.
3. Drizzle with maple syrup or honey if desired and sprinkle with cinnamon.

Avocado Toast with Tomato and Basil

Prep Time: 5 minutes Cook Time: 5 minutes (for toasting bread)
Serving Size: 2 slices

INGREDIENTS

1. 2 slices whole-grain bread (toasted)
2. 1 ripe avocado
6. Sea salt and black pepper to taste
3. 1 medium tomato (sliced)
4. Fresh basil leaves
5. Lemon juice

PREPARATION

1. Mash the ripe avocado with a fork and season with lemon juice, sea salt, and black pepper.
2. Spread the mashed avocado evenly on the toasted bread slices.
3. Top with sliced tomato and fresh basil leaves.

Chia Seed Pudding

Prep Time: 5 minutes   Cook Time: 0 minutes   Serving Size: 1 bowl

INGREDIENTS

1. 1/4 cup chia seeds
2. 1 cup almond milk or coconut milk
3. 1 tablespoon maple syrup or honey (optional)
4. Fresh fruit for topping (such as berries, sliced banana, or mango)
5. Nuts or seeds for topping (such as sliced almonds or hemp seeds)

PREPARATION

1. In a bowl, mix chia seeds and almond milk (or coconut milk) thoroughly.
2. Let the mixture sit for at least 30 minutes or refrigerate overnight, stirring occasionally

until it thickens into a pudding-like consistency.
3. Sweeten with maple syrup or honey if desired.

4. Serve topped with fresh fruit and nuts or seeds

Coconut Yogurt Parfait

Prep Time: 5 minutes   Cook Time: 0 minutes   Serving Size: 1 parfait

INGREDIENTS

1. 1 cup coconut yogurt
2. 1/2 cup mixed berries
3. 1/4 cup granola (choose a low-sugar, whole grain option)
4. 1 tablespoon shredded coconut

PREPARATION

1. In a glass or bowl, layer coconut yogurt, mixed berries, and granola.
2. Repeat layers until ingredients are used up.
3. Top with shredded coconut.

Lunch Ideas for Nourishing Meals

Quinoa Salad with Avocado and Chickpeas

Cook Time: 20 minutes Prep Time: 10 minutes Serving Size: 2-4

INGREDIENTS

Quinoa, avocado, chickpeas, cucumber, cherry tomatoes, red onion, lemon juice, olive oil, fresh herbs (such as parsley or cilantro), salt, pepper.

PREPARATION PROCESS

Cook quinoa according to package instructions. Chop vegetables and avocado. Mix cooked quinoa with vegetables, chickpeas, lemon juice, olive oil, herbs, salt, and pepper.

Grilled Vegetable Wrap

Cook Time: 15 minutes Prep Time: 10 minutes Serving Size: 2

INGREDIENTS

Whole grain tortillas, eggplant, zucchini, bell peppers, red onion, hummus, spinach leaves, balsamic vinegar, olive oil, salt, pepper.

PREPARATION PROCESS

Slice vegetables and grill until tender. Spread hummus on tortillas, add grilled vegetables and spinach leaves, drizzle with balsamic vinegar and olive oil, season with salt and pepper, and wrap.

Spinach and Lentil Salad

Cook Time: 10 minutes (for lentils) Prep Time: 15 minutes Serving Size: 2-3

INGREDIENTS

Spinach leaves, cooked lentils, cherry tomatoes, cucumber, red onion, bell pepper, avocado, lemon juice, olive oil, garlic, salt, pepper.

PREPARATION PROCESS

Combine spinach, cooked lentils, chopped vegetables, and avocado. Make a dressing with lemon juice, olive oil, minced garlic, salt, and pepper. Toss salad with dressing.

Mediterranean Chickpea Salad

Cook Time: 5 minutes (if using canned chickpeas) Prep Time: 15 minutes Serving Size: 2-3

INGREDIENTS

Cooked chickpeas, cherry tomatoes, cucumber, red onion, Kalamata olives, parsley, lemon juice, olive oil, garlic, salt, pepper.

PREPARATION PROCESS

Combine chickpeas, chopped vegetables, olives, and parsley. Make a dressing with lemon juice, olive oil, minced garlic, salt, and pepper. Toss salad with dressing.

Stuffed Bell Peppers with Quinoa and Black Beans

Cook Time: 30 minutes Prep Time: 20 minutes Serving Size: 4

INGREDIENTS

Bell peppers, cooked quinoa, black beans, corn, onion, garlic, tomato sauce, cumin, paprika, chili powder, salt, pepper, vegan cheese (optional).

PREPARATION PROCESS

Cut tops off bell peppers and remove seeds. Saute onion and garlic, then mix with cooked quinoa, black beans, corn, tomato sauce, and spices. Stuff peppers with quinoa mixture, top with vegan cheese if desired, and bake until peppers are tender.

Lentil and Vegetable Soup

Cook Time: 30 minutes Prep Time: 15 minutes Serving Size: 4-6

INGREDIENTS

Lentils, carrots, celery, onion, garlic, vegetable broth, tomatoes, spinach, thyme, bay leaves, salt, pepper.

PREPARATION PROCESS

Saute onion, garlic, carrots, and celery until softened. Add lentils, tomatoes, vegetable broth, thyme, bay leaves, salt, and pepper. Simmer until lentils are tender. Stir in spinach before serving.

Zucchini Noodles with Pesto and Cherry Tomatoes

Cook Time: 10 minutes Prep Time: 15 minutes Serving Size: 2

INGREDIENTS

Zucchini, cherry tomatoes, basil, garlic, pine nuts, nutritional yeast, olive oil, lemon juice, salt, pepper.

PREPARATION PROCESS

Spiralize zucchini into noodles. Blend basil, garlic, pine nuts, nutritional yeast, olive oil, lemon juice, salt, and pepper to make pesto. Toss zucchini noodles with pesto and cherry tomatoes

Chickpea and Vegetable Stir-Fry

Cook Time: 20 minutes Prep Time: 15 minutes Serving Size: 4

INGREDIENTS

Cooked chickpeas, broccoli, bell peppers, snap peas, carrots, onion, garlic, ginger, soy sauce (or tamari), sesame oil, rice vinegar, maple syrup, cornstarch, water, sesame seeds, green onions.

PREPARATION PROCESS

Stir-fry vegetables, garlic, and ginger in sesame oil until tender-crisp. Add cooked chickpeas. Mix soy sauce, rice vinegar, maple syrup, cornstarch, and water to make a sauce. Pour sauce over stir-fry and cook until thickened. Serve over rice or quinoa, garnished with sesame seeds and green onions.

Sweet Potato and Black Bean Buddha Bowl

Cook Time: 15 minutes Prep Time: 15 minutes Serving Size: 4

INGREDIENTS

Roasted sweet potatoes, cooked black beans, quinoa, avocado, kale, red cabbage, radishes, tahini dressing (tahini, lemon juice, garlic, water, salt).

PREPARATION PROCESS

Arrange roasted sweet potatoes, cooked black beans, quinoa, sliced avocado, kale, shredded red cabbage, and sliced radishes in bowls. Drizzle with tahini dressing.

Cauliflower Rice Stir-Fry

INGREDIENTS

Cauliflower, bell peppers, broccoli, carrots, snap peas, onion, garlic, ginger, soy sauce (or tamari), sesame oil, rice vinegar, maple syrup, cornstarch, water, green onions.

PREPARATION PROCESS

Pulse cauliflower in a food processor to make rice-like texture. Stir-fry vegetables, garlic, and ginger in sesame oil until tender-crisp. Add cauliflower rice. Mix soy sauce, rice vinegar, maple syrup, cornstarch, and water to make a sauce. Pour sauce over stir-fry and cook until thickened. Serve garnished with sliced green onions.

Dinner Recipes for Flavorful and Nutritious Entrees

Quinoa-Stuffed Bell Peppers

Prep Time: 15 minutes Cook Time: 30 minutes Serving Size: 2 stuffed peppers

INGREDIENTS

Bell peppers, quinoa, black beans, diced tomatoes, onions, garlic, spinach, vegetable broth, cumin, paprika, salt, pepper.

PREPARATION

Preheat oven. Cook quinoa. Sauté onions and garlic, then add spinach and seasonings. Combine with cooked quinoa and black beans. Stuff mixture into halved bell peppers. Bake until peppers are tender.

Baked Lemon Herb Salmon

Prep Time: 10 minutes Cook Time: 15 minutes Serving Size: 1 fillet

INGREDIENTS

Salmon fillets, lemon, garlic, fresh herbs (such as parsley, dill, and thyme), olive oil, salt, pepper.

PREPARATION

Preheat oven. Place salmon fillets on a baking sheet. Drizzle with olive oil, lemon juice, and minced garlic. Sprinkle with fresh herbs, salt, and pepper. Bake until salmon is cooked through.

Mushroom and Spinach Stir-Fry

Prep Time: 10 minutes Cook Time: 15 minutes Serving Size: 2 cups

INGREDIENTS

Mushrooms, spinach, bell peppers, onions, garlic, ginger, tamari sauce (or soy sauce), sesame oil, rice vinegar.

PREPARATION

Sauté onions, garlic, and ginger. Add sliced mushrooms and bell peppers, cook until tender. Add spinach and stir in tamari sauce and rice vinegar. Serve hot.

Zucchini Noodles with Avocado Pesto

Prep Time: 15 minutes Cook Time: 0 minutes Serving Size: 2 cups

INGREDIENTS

Zucchini, avocado, basil, garlic, lemon juice, pine nuts, olive oil, salt, pepper.

PREPARATION

Spiralize zucchini into noodles. Blend avocado, basil, garlic, lemon juice, pine nuts, and olive oil until smooth. Toss zucchini noodles with avocado pesto. Serve chilled or lightly warmed.

Chickpea and Vegetable Curry

Prep Time: 15 minutes Cook Time: 20 minutes Serving Size: 1 cup

INGREDIENTS

Chickpeas, coconut milk, tomatoes, onions, garlic, ginger, curry powder, turmeric, cumin, coriander, spinach, cilantro.

PREPARATION

Sauté onions, garlic, and ginger. Add diced tomatoes and coconut milk, then stir in spices. Add chickpeas and simmer until flavors meld. Stir in spinach and cilantro before serving.

Grilled Portobello Mushroom Steaks

Prep Time: 10 minutes Cook Time: 10 minutes Serving Size: 1 mushroom

INGREDIENTS

Portobello mushrooms, balsamic vinegar, olive oil, garlic, thyme, rosemary, salt, pepper.

PREPARATION

Marinate mushrooms in balsamic vinegar, olive oil, minced garlic, and herbs. Grill until tender and lightly charred.

Lentil and Vegetable Soup

Prep Time: 15 minutes Cook Time: 30 minutes Serving Size: 1.5 cups

INGREDIENTS

Lentils, carrots, celery, onions, garlic, tomatoes, vegetable broth, spinach, thyme, bay leaves, salt, pepper.

PREPARATION

Sauté onions, garlic, carrots, and celery. Add lentils, diced tomatoes, vegetable broth, and seasonings. Simmer until lentils are tender. Stir in spinach before serving.

Baked Stuffed Sweet Potatoes

Prep Time: 15 minutes Cook Time: 45 minutes Serving Size: 1 stuffed sweet potato

INGREDIENTS

Sweet potatoes, black beans, corn, red bell pepper, onions, garlic, cumin, chili powder, cilantro, lime juice, salt, pepper.

PREPARATION

Bake sweet potatoes until tender. Sauté onions, garlic, and bell pepper. Add black beans, corn, and seasonings. Stuff mixture into baked sweet potatoes. Garnish with cilantro and lime juice.

Cauliflower Fried Rice

Prep Time: 10 minutes Cook Time: 15 minutes Serving Size: 1 cup

INGREDIENTS

Cauliflower rice, mixed vegetables (such as peas, carrots, and bell peppers), onions, garlic, ginger, tamari sauce (or soy sauce), sesame oil, green onions.

PREPARATION

Sauté onions, garlic, and ginger. Add mixed vegetables and cauliflower rice, cook until tender. Stir in tamari sauce and sesame oil. Garnish with chopped green onions.

Baked Eggplant Parmesan

Prep Time: 20 minutes Cook Time: 30 minutes Serving Size: 1/2 eggplant

INGREDIENTS

Eggplant, whole wheat breadcrumbs, marinara sauce, mozzarella cheese, Parmesan cheese, basil, olive oil, salt, pepper.

PREPARATION

Slice eggplant, dip in beaten egg, then coat with breadcrumbs. Bake until golden and crispy. Layer with marinara sauce, mozzarella, and Parmesan cheese. Bake until cheese is bubbly. Garnish with fresh basil.

Snacks and Side Dishes to Support Your Alkaline Journey

Avocado and Tomato Salad

Prep Time: 10 minutes Cook Time: 0 minutes Serving Size: 2

INGREDIENTS

Avocado, tomatoes, red onion, cucumber, lemon juice, olive oil, fresh basil leaves, sea salt, black pepper.

PREPARATION

Chop avocado, tomatoes, red onion, and cucumber into bite-sized pieces. Combine in a bowl with lemon juice, olive oil, chopped basil leaves, sea salt, and black pepper.

Cucumber and Carrot Sticks with Hummus

Prep Time: 5 minutes Cook Time: 0 minutes Serving Size: 2

INGREDIENTS

Cucumber, carrots, hummus (store-bought or homemade).

PREPARATION

Wash and slice cucumber and carrots into sticks. Serve with hummus for dipping.

Quinoa Salad with Chickpeas and Spinach

Prep Time: 15 minutes Cook Time: 15 minutes (for quinoa) Serving Size: 4

INGREDIENTS

Quinoa, chickpeas, spinach, cherry tomatoes, red bell pepper, lemon juice, olive oil, garlic, sea salt, black pepper.

PREPARATION

Cook quinoa according to package instructions. Mix cooked quinoa with drained and rinsed chickpeas, chopped spinach, halved cherry tomatoes, diced red bell pepper, lemon juice, olive oil, minced garlic, sea salt, and black pepper.

Zucchini Noodles with Pesto

Prep Time: 15 minutes Cook Time: 0 minutes Serving Size: 2

INGREDIENTS

Zucchini, fresh basil leaves, pine nuts, garlic, lemon juice, nutritional yeast, olive oil, sea salt, black pepper.

PREPARATION

Use a spiralizer to create zucchini noodles. In a food processor, blend fresh basil leaves, pine nuts, garlic, lemon juice, nutritional yeast, olive oil, sea salt, and black pepper to make pesto. Toss zucchini noodles with pesto sauce.

Stuffed Bell Peppers

Prep Time: 20 minutes Cook Time: 30 minutes Serving Size: 4

INGREDIENTS

Bell peppers, quinoa, black beans, corn, tomatoes, onion, garlic, cumin, chili powder, avocado, lime, cilantro, sea salt, black pepper.

PREPARATION

Cook quinoa according to package instructions. In a skillet, sauté onion and garlic until soft. Add cooked quinoa, black beans, corn, diced tomatoes, cumin, chili powder, sea salt, and black pepper. Cut bell peppers in half, remove seeds, and stuff with quinoa mixture. Bake in the oven until peppers are tender. Serve with sliced avocado, lime wedges, and chopped cilantro.

Kale Chips

Prep Time: 10 minutes Cook Time: 15-20 minutes Serving Size: 2

INGREDIENTS

Kale, olive oil, nutritional yeast, sea salt, black pepper.

PREPARATION

Preheat oven to 350°F (175°C). Wash and dry kale leaves, then tear into bite-sized pieces, removing tough stems. Massage kale with olive oil, nutritional yeast, sea salt, and black pepper. Spread out on a baking sheet and bake until crispy, about 15-20 minutes.

Sliced Apple with Almond Butter

Prep Time: 5 minutes Cook Time: 0 minutes Serving Size: 2

INGREDIENTS

Apples, almond butter.

PREPARATION

Wash and slice apples. Serve with almond butter for dipping.

Stuffed Mushrooms

Prep Time: 20 minutes Cook Time: 20 minutes Serving Size: 4

INGREDIENTS

Mushrooms, quinoa, spinach, onion, garlic, nutritional yeast, olive oil, sea salt, black pepper.

PREPARATION

Cook quinoa according to package instructions. In a skillet, sauté onion and garlic until soft. Add chopped spinach and cook until wilted. Mix cooked quinoa with sautéed vegetables, nutritional yeast, olive oil, sea salt, and black pepper. Stuff mushroom caps with quinoa mixture. Bake in the oven until mushrooms are tender.

Cucumber Tomato Salad

Prep Time: 10 minutes Cook Time: 0 minutes Serving Size: 2

INGREDIENTS

Cucumber, tomatoes, red onion, lemon juice, olive oil, fresh parsley, sea salt, black pepper.

PREPARATION

Chop cucumber, tomatoes, and red onion into bite-sized pieces. Combine in a bowl with lemon juice, olive oil, chopped parsley, sea salt, and black pepper.

Bean Salad

Prep Time: 15 minutes Cook Time: 0 minutes Serving Size: 4

INGREDIENTS

Mixed beans (such as kidney beans, black beans, chickpeas), bell pepper, cucumber, red onion, parsley, olive oil, lemon juice, garlic, sea salt, black pepper.

PREPARATION

Rinse and drain mixed beans. Chop bell pepper, cucumber, red onion, and parsley. Mix together in a bowl with beans, olive oil, lemon juice, minced garlic, sea salt, and black pepper.

Desserts and Treats for Indulgence Without Compromise

Alkaline Berry Smoothie Bowl

Cook Time: 5 minutes Prep Time: 5 minutes Serving Size: 1 bowl

INGREDIENTS

Mixed berries (strawberries, blueberries, raspberries), spinach, banana, almond milk, chia seeds.

PREPARATION

Blend mixed berries, spinach, banana, and almond milk until smooth. Pour into a bowl and top with chia seeds.

Chia Seed Pudding

Cook Time: 0 minutes Prep Time: 5 minutes (+ chilling time) Serving Size: 1 bowl

INGREDIENTS

Chia seeds, almond milk, vanilla extract, maple syrup, mixed berries.

PREPARATION

Mix chia seeds, almond milk, vanilla extract, and maple syrup in a bowl. Let it sit in the fridge for at least 2 hours or overnight. Serve with mixed berries on top.

Almond Butter Banana Bites

Cook Time: 0 minutes Prep Time: 10 minutes Serving Size: Varies

INGREDIENTS

Bananas, almond butter, unsweetened shredded coconut, cacao nibs.

PREPARATION

Slice bananas into rounds. Spread almond butter on each banana slice and sprinkle with shredded coconut and cacao nibs.

Avocado Chocolate Mousse

Cook Time: 0 minutes Prep Time: 10 minutes Serving Size: Varies

INGREDIENTS

Avocado, cocoa powder, maple syrup, vanilla extract, almond milk.

PREPARATION

Blend avocado, cocoa powder, maple syrup, vanilla extract, and almond milk until smooth and creamy. Chill in the fridge before serving.

Coconut Matcha Energy Balls

Cook Time: 0 minutes Prep Time: 15 minutes Serving Size: Varies

INGREDIENTS

Dates, almonds, shredded coconut, matcha powder, lemon zest.

PREPARATION

Blend dates, almonds, shredded coconut, matcha powder, and lemon zest in a food processor until sticky. Roll into balls and refrigerate until firm.

Turmeric Golden Milk Popsicles

Cook Time: 0 minutes Prep Time: 5 minutes (+ freezing time) Serving Size: Varies

INGREDIENTS

Coconut milk, turmeric powder, ginger powder, cinnamon, black pepper, honey.

Mix coconut milk, turmeric powder, ginger powder, cinnamon, black pepper, and honey in a bowl. Pour into popsicle molds and freeze until solid.

PREPARATION

Raw Lemon Coconut Bars

Cook Time: 0 minutes Prep Time: 15 minutes (+ chilling time)
Serving Size: Varies

INGREDIENTS

Almonds, dates, shredded coconut, lemon juice, lemon zest.

PREPARATION

Blend almonds, dates, shredded coconut, lemon juice, and lemon zest in a food processor until sticky. Press into a pan and refrigerate until firm. Cut into bars before serving.

Blueberry Almond Oat Bars

Cook Time: 25 minutes Prep Time: 15 minutes Serving Size: Varies

INGREDIENTS

Oats, almonds, dates, blueberries, almond butter, maple syrup.

PREPARATION

Blend oats, almonds, and dates in a food processor. Press half of the mixture into a pan. Mix blueberries, almond butter, and maple syrup in a bowl and spread over the oat mixture. Crumble the remaining oat mixture on top. Bake in the oven until golden brown.

Watermelon Mint Sorbet

Cook Time: 0 minutes Prep Time: 10 minutes (+ freezing time)
Serving Size: Varies

INGREDIENTS

Watermelon, fresh mint leaves, lime juice, honey.

PREPARATION

Blend watermelon, fresh mint leaves, lime juice, and honey until smooth. Pour into a shallow dish and freeze until firm. Scrape with a fork to create a sorbet texture.

Mixed Berry Frozen Yogurt Bark

Cook Time: 0 minutes Prep Time: 5 minutes (+ freezing time)
Serving Size: Varies

INGREDIENTS

Greek yogurt, mixed berries (strawberries, blueberries, raspberries), honey.

PREPARATION

Mix Greek yogurt and honey in a bowl. Spread onto a baking sheet lined with parchment paper. Sprinkle mixed berries on top and freeze until firm. Break into pieces before serving.

Mediterranean Alkaline Recipes

Mediterranean Quinoa Salad

Prep Time: 15 minutes Cook Time: 15 minutes Serving Size: 4

INGREDIENTS

Quinoa, cherry tomatoes, cucumbers, bell peppers, red onion, Kalamata olives, fresh parsley, lemon juice, olive oil, salt, pepper.

PREPARATION PROCESS

Cook quinoa according to package instructions. Chop vegetables and herbs. Combine all ingredients in a large bowl and toss with lemon juice, olive oil, salt, and pepper.

Grilled Mediterranean Vegetable Skewers

Prep Time: 20 minutes Cook Time: 15 minutes Serving Size: 4

INGREDIENTS

Zucchini, eggplant, bell peppers, cherry tomatoes, red onion, button mushrooms, olive oil, lemon juice, garlic, oregano, salt, pepper.

PREPARATION PROCESS

Cut vegetables into chunks. Marinate in olive oil, lemon juice, garlic, oregano, salt, and pepper. Thread onto skewers and grill until tender.

Mediterranean Chickpea Salad

Prep Time: 15 minutes   Serving Size: 4

INGREDIENTS

Chickpeas, cherry tomatoes, cucumbers, red onion, Kalamata olives, feta cheese (optional), fresh parsley, olive oil, lemon juice, garlic, oregano, salt, pepper.

PREPARATION PROCESS

Rinse and drain chickpeas. Chop vegetables and herbs. Combine all ingredients in a bowl and toss with olive oil, lemon juice, garlic, oregano, salt, and pepper.

Baked Mediterranean Stuffed Peppers

Prep Time: 20 minutes Cook Time: 25 minutes Serving Size: 4

INGREDIENTS

Bell peppers, quinoa, chickpeas, cherry tomatoes, spinach, red onion, garlic, feta cheese (optional), olive oil, lemon juice, oregano, salt, pepper.

PREPARATION PROCESS

Cook quinoa according to package instructions. Sauté garlic, onion, and spinach. Mix with quinoa, chickpeas, tomatoes, feta cheese, olive oil, lemon juice, oregano, salt, and pepper. Stuff peppers and bake until tender.

Mediterranean Lentil Soup

Prep Time: 15 minutes Cook Time: 30 minutes Serving Size: 6

INGREDIENTS

Lentils, carrots, celery, onion, garlic, tomatoes, vegetable broth, olive oil, lemon juice, cumin, coriander, turmeric, salt, pepper.

PREPARATION PROCESS

Sauté onion, garlic, carrots, and celery. Add lentils, tomatoes, vegetable broth, and spices. Simmer until lentils are tender. Finish with olive oil and lemon juice.

Mediterranean Grilled Eggplant with Tahini Sauce

Prep Time: 15 minutes Cook Time: 10 minutes Serving Size: 4

INGREDIENTS

Eggplant, olive oil, garlic, lemon juice, tahini, water, parsley, cumin, salt, pepper.

PREPARATION PROCESS

Slice eggplant and brush with olive oil. Grill until tender. Prepare tahini sauce by mixing tahini, lemon juice, water, garlic, parsley, cumin, salt, and pepper. Drizzle over grilled eggplant.

Mediterranean Roasted Beet Salad

Prep Time: 15 minutes Cook Time: 45 minutes Serving Size: 4

INGREDIENTS

Beets, arugula, oranges, red onion, feta cheese (optional), balsamic vinegar, olive oil, honey, Dijon mustard, salt, pepper.

PREPARATION PROCESS

Roast beets until tender. Peel and slice. Arrange on a bed of arugula with orange segments, sliced onion, and crumbled feta cheese. Whisk together balsamic vinaigrette and drizzle over salad.

Mediterranean Cauliflower Rice Pilaf

Prep Time: 20 minutes Cook Time: 15 minutes Serving Size: 4

INGREDIENTS

Cauliflower, cherry tomatoes, bell peppers, red onion, garlic, olives, parsley, lemon juice, olive oil, cumin, coriander, salt, pepper.

PREPARATION PROCESS

Pulse cauliflower in a food processor to rice-like consistency. Sauté garlic, onion, and peppers. Add cauliflower rice, tomatoes, olives, parsley, lemon juice, and spices. Cook until tender.

Mediterranean Grilled Swordfish with Lemon-Herb Marinade

Prep Time: 10 minutes Cook Time: 10 minutes Serving Size: 4

INGREDIENTS

Swordfish steaks, lemon zest, lemon juice, garlic, fresh herbs (such as parsley, oregano, thyme), olive oil, salt, pepper.

PREPARATION PROCESS

Prepare marinade by combining lemon zest, lemon juice, minced garlic, chopped herbs, olive oil, salt, and pepper. Marinate swordfish steaks for 30 minutes. Grill until cooked through.

Mediterranean Roasted Vegetable Tart

Prep Time: 20 minutes Cook Time: 25 minutes Serving Size: 6

INGREDIENTS

Puff pastry, eggplant, zucchini, bell peppers, cherry tomatoes, red onion, garlic, olive oil, fresh herbs (such as thyme, rosemary), salt, pepper.

PREPARATION PROCESS

Roll out puff pastry and place on a baking sheet. Arrange sliced vegetables on top, drizzle with olive oil, sprinkle with minced garlic, herbs, salt, and pepper. Bake until pastry is golden and vegetables are tender.

Chapter 4

Meal Planning and Preparation

Weekly Meal Plans and Shopping Lists

30 DAY MEAL PLAN

DAY	BREAKFAST	LUNCH	DINNER
1	Green Smoothie Bowl	Quinoa Salad with Avocado and Chickpeas	Quinoa-Stuffed Bell Peppers
2	Quinoa Breakfast Bowl	Grilled Vegetable Wrap	Baked Lemon Herb Salmon
3	Avocado Toast with Tomato and Basil	Spinach and Lentil Salad	Mushroom and Spinach Stir-Fry
4	Chia Seed Pudding	Mediterranean Chickpea Salad	Zucchini Noodles with Avocado Pesto
5	Coconut Yogurt Parfait	Stuffed Bell Peppers with Quinoa and Black Beans	Cauliflower Fried Rice
6	Alkaline Berry Smoothie Bowl	Lentil and Vegetable Soup	Baked Stuffed Sweet Potatoes
7	Quinoa Breakfast Bowl	Chickpea and Vegetable Stir-Fry	Grilled Portobello Mushroom Steaks

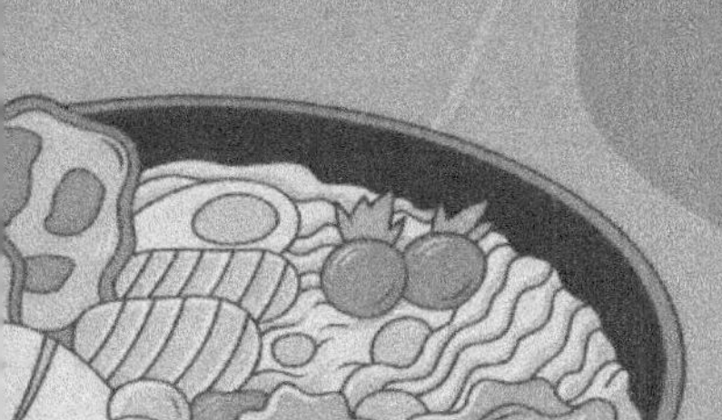
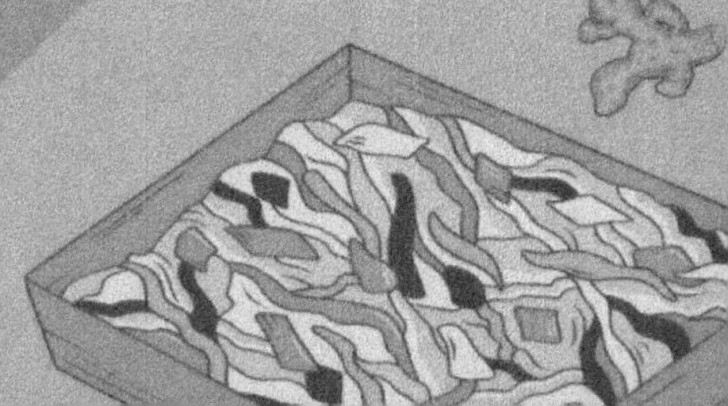

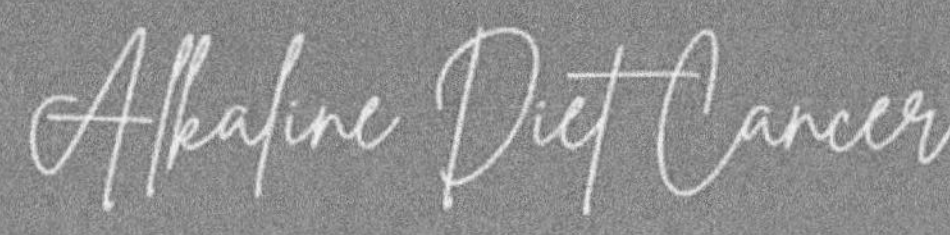

30 DAY MEAL PLAN

DAY	BREAKFAST	LUNCH	DINNER
8	Green Smoothie Bowl	Mediterranean Chickpea Salad	Quinoa-Stuffed Bell Peppers
9	Chia Seed Pudding	Zucchini Noodles with Pesto and Cherry Tomatoes	Baked Lemon Herb Salmon
10	Avocado Toast with Tomato and Basil	Lentil and Vegetable Soup	Stuffed Bell Peppers with Quinoa and Black Beans
11	Coconut Yogurt Parfait	Grilled Vegetable Wrap	Mushroom and Spinach Stir-Fry
12	Almond Butter Banana Bites	Quinoa Salad with Avocado and Chickpeas	Cauliflower Fried Rice
13	Green Smoothie Bowl	Spinach and Lentil Salad	Baked Stuffed Sweet Potatoes
14	Quinoa Breakfast Bowl	Mediterranean Chickpea Salad	Zucchini Noodles with Avocado Pesto

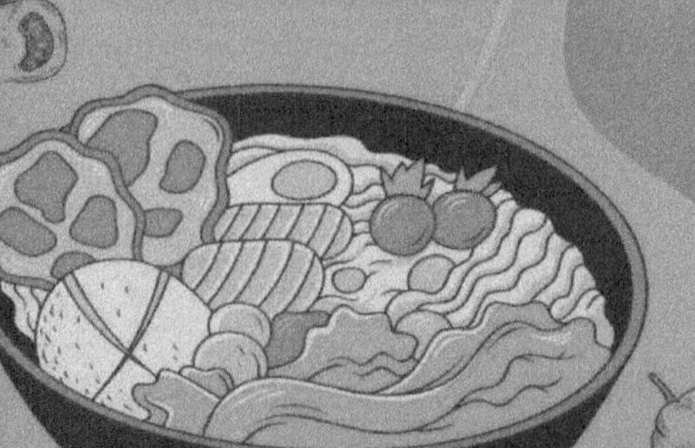
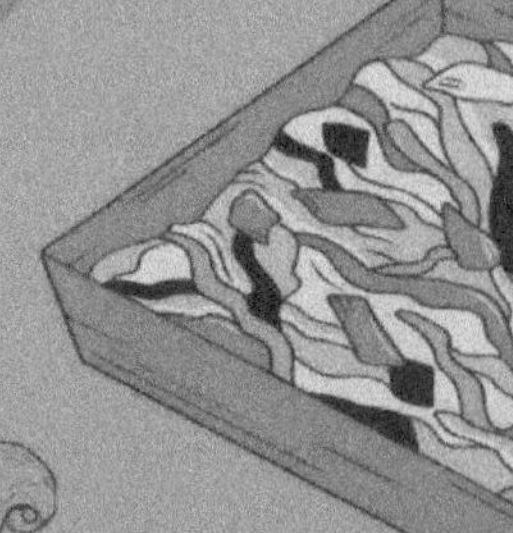

30 DAY MEAL PLAN

DAY	BREAKFAST	LUNCH	DINNER
15	Chia Seed Pudding	Stuffed Bell Peppers with Quinoa and Black Beans	Grilled Portobello Mushroom Steaks
16	Avocado Toast with Tomato and Basil	Chickpea and Vegetable Stir-Fry	Baked Lemon Herb Salmon
17	Coconut Yogurt Parfait	Lentil and Vegetable Soup	Mushroom and Spinach Stir-Fry
18	Alkaline Berry Smoothie Bowl	Grilled Vegetable Wrap	Quinoa-Stuffed Bell Peppers
19	Quinoa Breakfast Bowl	Mediterranean Chickpea Salad	Cauliflower Fried Rice
20	Green Smoothie Bowl	Spinach and Lentil Salad	Baked Stuffed Sweet Potatoes
21	Chia Seed Pudding	Zucchini Noodles with Pesto and Cherry Tomatoes	Grilled Portobello Mushroom Steaks
22	Avocado Toast with Tomato and Basil	Stuffed Bell Peppers with Quinoa and Black Beans	Quinoa-Stuffed Bell Peppers

Alkaline Diet Cancer
30 DAY MEAL PLAN

DAY	BREAKFAST	LUNCH	DINNER
23	Green Smoothie Bowl	Chickpea and Vegetable Stir-Fry	Baked Lemon Herb Salmon
24	Coconut Yogurt Parfait	Lentil and Vegetable Soup	Mushroom and Spinach Stir-Fry
25	Almond Butter Banana Bites	Quinoa Salad with Avocado and Chickpeas	Cauliflower Fried Rice
26	Quinoa Breakfast Bowl	Mediterranean Chickpea Salad	Zucchini Noodles with Avocado Pesto
27	Chia Seed Pudding	Stuffed Bell Peppers with Quinoa and Black Beans	Grilled Portobello Mushroom Steaks
28	Avocado Toast with Tomato and Basil	Chickpea and Vegetable Stir-Fry	Baked Lemon Herb Salmon
29	Coconut Yogurt Parfait	Lentil and Vegetable Soup	Mushroom and Spinach Stir-Fry
30	Alkaline Berry Smoothie Bowl	Quinoa Salad with Avocado and Chickpeas	Stuffed Bell Peppers with Quinoa and Black Beans

Chapter 5

Lifestyle Strategies for Cancer Prevention

Cancer is a complex illness that is influenced by a number of genetic, environmental, and lifestyle variables. A person's chance of acquiring cancer may be considerably decreased by implementing certain lifestyle measures, even when certain risk factors, such as age and family history, cannot be changed. These tactics help reduce the occurrence of cancer in addition to enhancing general health and wellbeing.

Keeping a Healthy Weight: Overweight and obesity are linked to a higher risk of developing breast, colon, and pancreatic cancers, among other cancers. This risk may be decreased by aiming for a healthy weight via a balanced diet and frequent exercise.

Consuming an Equitable Diet: Antioxidants and other vital nutrients found in a diet rich in fruits, vegetables, whole grains, and lean proteins help shield cells from oxidative damage that may cause cancer. Including a range of vibrant fruits and vegetables guarantees a varied diet of antioxidant-rich vitamins, minerals, and phytochemicals.

Frequent Moderate to Vigorous Physical Exercise: Maintaining a healthy weight is made easier by frequent moderate to vigorous physical exercise, which also lowers the chance of acquiring certain malignancies, including endometrial, breast, and colon cancer. Aim for 150 minutes or more of moderate-to-intense activity per week or 75 minutes or more of strenuous exercise.

Reducing Alcohol Consumption: Drinking alcohol has been associated with a higher risk of breast, liver, and colon cancers, among other cancers. Reducing alcohol use or giving it up completely may lower the risk of developing some malignancies.

Steer clear of tobacco products. Using tobacco is one of the main causes of cancer globally and contributes significantly to the death toll from the disease. Preventing cancer requires abstaining from all tobacco products, including smoking and chewing tobacco.

Preventing Sun Exposure: Skin cancer, including melanoma, is one of the most avoidable forms of cancer. Seek shade, put on protective clothes, use sunscreen with a high SPF, stay away from tanning beds and sunlamps, and protect your skin.

Getting Vaccinated: Hepatitis B and human papillomavirus (HPV) infections are linked to a higher risk of liver cancer and cervical cancer, respectively. Immunization against these viruses may aid in the prevention of associated malignancies.

Frequent Screening and Early Detection: The results of cancer therapy may be greatly enhanced by early detection obtained by routine screenings, such as mammograms, Pap smears, colonoscopies, and prostate examinations. Observe the screening recommendations made in accordance with your age, gender, and personal risk factors.

Handling stress: Prolonged stress may impair immunity and encourage inflammation, both of which can hasten the onset of cancer. These effects may be lessened by using stress-reduction practices including yoga, meditation, mindfulness, and deep breathing exercises.

Encouraging Sound Sleep Practices: Breast and colorectal cancer risk are among the malignancies that are linked to poor sleep quality and inadequate sleep. By adopting a regular sleep routine and providing a peaceful sleeping environment, aim for 7-9 hours of excellent sleep every night.

By incorporating these lifestyle recommendations into your daily routine, you can lower your cancer risk and improve your general health and well-being. Making wise decisions and prioritizing cancer prevention habits throughout life is critical.

Conclusion

As it comes to an end, "The Alkaline Diet Cancer Cookbook for Beginners" provides more than simply a list of recipes—rather, it provides a whole manual for embracing a way of life centered on vitality, health, and cancer prevention. During this trip, readers have explored the principles of the alkaline diet and its ability to restore the body's pH balance and create an environment that is less favorable to cancer development.

Readers have found tasty and nutritious recipes made with carefully chosen ingredients to promote cellular health and alkalinity at every turn of the page. The wide range of recipes shows that following an alkaline diet can be tasty and fulfilling. From vibrant smoothie bowls to filling quinoa salads and substantial main courses,

This cookbook has proven to be a valuable resource for understanding the complex relationship between nutrition, lifestyle, and cancer prevention, going beyond the area of culinary experimentation. Through conversations on the importance of maintaining a healthy weight, getting regular exercise, and making thoughtful decisions regarding alcohol and tobacco use, readers have learned important information about all-encompassing strategies for lowering the risk of cancer.

As we get to the end of this cookbook, let's not see it as just the end of a journey through food but rather as the start of a whole new way of living. Equipped with information, motivation, and an abundance of nutritious recipes, readers are enabled to set out on a journey toward achieving their utmost health and wellness.

May the ideas and methods discussed in these pages, which are centered on empowerment and resiliency, be a source of inspiration and direction for everyone aiming to avoid cancer and have a healthy life. Allow this cookbook to serve as a guide on the path to long-term health and pleasure, not simply a handy reference in the kitchen.

Acknowledgments

I would like to express my heartfelt gratitude to the following individuals for their invaluable support and contributions to this book:

- My family, for their unwavering encouragement and belief in my endeavors.
- My friends, for their inspiration and enthusiasm throughout this journey.
- The dedicated team at the publishing house, for their expertise and guidance in bringing this book to fruition.
- The readers, whose curiosity and passion for health and wellness continue to inspire me every day.

Thank you for being a part of this journey.

Additional Resources
Recommended Reading and References

Balancing pH Levels Deliciously: An Easy-to-Follow Acid-Alkaline Diet Cookbook for Beginners

Alkaline Diet Cancer Cookbook For Beginners : A Comprehensive Guide to the Alkaline Diet's Transformative Power for Optimal Health, Inflammation Reduction

Alkaline diet cookbook for diabetes: 150 Alkaline Recipes to prevent and reverse diabetes, and Bring Your Body Back to Balance

Get our new free Ebook by scanning the QR Code Below

WEEKLY MEAL PLANNING

Month: ______________
Week:
(1) (2) (3) (4)

Sunday

Breakfast: ______________

Calories	Protein	Sugar	Carbs

Lunch: ______________

Calories	Protein	Sugar	Carbs

Dinner: ______________

Calories	Protein	Sugar	Carbs

Monday

Breakfast: ______________

Calories	Protein	Sugar	Carbs

Lunch: ______________

Calories	Protein	Sugar	Carbs

Dinner: ______________

Calories	Protein	Sugar	Carbs

Tuesday

Breakfast: ______________

Calories	Protein	Sugar	Carbs

Lunch: ______________

Calories	Protein	Sugar	Carbs

Dinner: ______________

Calories	Protein	Sugar	Carbs

Wednesday

Breakfast: ______________

Calories	Protein	Sugar	Carbs

Lunch: ______________

Calories	Protein	Sugar	Carbs

Dinner: ______________

Calories	Protein	Sugar	Carbs

Thursday

Breakfast: ______________

Calories	Protein	Sugar	Carbs

Lunch: ______________

Calories	Protein	Sugar	Carbs

Dinner: ______________

Calories	Protein	Sugar	Carbs

Friday

Breakfast: ______________

Calories	Protein	Sugar	Carbs

Lunch: ______________

Calories	Protein	Sugar	Carbs

Dinner: ______________

Calories	Protein	Sugar	Carbs

Saturday

Breakfast: ______________

Calories	Protein	Sugar	Carbs

Lunch: ______________

Calories	Protein	Sugar	Carbs

Dinner: ______________

Calories	Protein	Sugar	Carbs

Shopping List:

WEEKLY MEAL PLANNING

Month: ___________

Week:

(1) (2) (3) (4)

Sunday

Breakfast: __________

Calories	Protein	Sugar	Carbs

Lunch: __________

Calories	Protein	Sugar	Carbs

Dinner: __________

Calories	Protein	Sugar	Carbs

Monday

Breakfast: __________

Calories	Protein	Sugar	Carbs

Lunch: __________

Calories	Protein	Sugar	Carbs

Dinner: __________

Calories	Protein	Sugar	Carbs

Tuesday

Breakfast: __________

Calories	Protein	Sugar	Carbs

Lunch: __________

Calories	Protein	Sugar	Carbs

Dinner: __________

Calories	Protein	Sugar	Carbs

Wednesday

Breakfast: __________

Calories	Protein	Sugar	Carbs

Lunch: __________

Calories	Protein	Sugar	Carbs

Dinner: __________

Calories	Protein	Sugar	Carbs

Thursday

Breakfast: __________

Calories	Protein	Sugar	Carbs

Lunch: __________

Calories	Protein	Sugar	Carbs

Dinner: __________

Calories	Protein	Sugar	Carbs

Friday

Breakfast: __________

Calories	Protein	Sugar	Carbs

Lunch: __________

Calories	Protein	Sugar	Carbs

Dinner: __________

Calories	Protein	Sugar	Carbs

Saturday

Breakfast: __________

Calories	Protein	Sugar	Carbs

Lunch: __________

Calories	Protein	Sugar	Carbs

Dinner: __________

Calories	Protein	Sugar	Carbs

Shopping List:

WEEKLY MEAL PLANNING

Month: ___________

Week:

(1) (2) (3) (4)

Sunday

Breakfast: ___________

Calories	Protein	Sugar	Carbs

Lunch: ___________

Calories	Protein	Sugar	Carbs

Dinner: ___________

Calories	Protein	Sugar	Carbs

Monday

Breakfast: ___________

Calories	Protein	Sugar	Carbs

Lunch: ___________

Calories	Protein	Sugar	Carbs

Dinner: ___________

Calories	Protein	Sugar	Carbs

Tuesday

Breakfast: ___________

Calories	Protein	Sugar	Carbs

Lunch: ___________

Calories	Protein	Sugar	Carbs

Dinner: ___________

Calories	Protein	Sugar	Carbs

Wednesday

Breakfast: ___________

Calories	Protein	Sugar	Carbs

Lunch: ___________

Calories	Protein	Sugar	Carbs

Dinner: ___________

Calories	Protein	Sugar	Carbs

Thursday

Breakfast: ___________

Calories	Protein	Sugar	Carbs

Lunch: ___________

Calories	Protein	Sugar	Carbs

Dinner: ___________

Calories	Protein	Sugar	Carbs

Friday

Breakfast: ___________

Calories	Protein	Sugar	Carbs

Lunch: ___________

Calories	Protein	Sugar	Carbs

Dinner: ___________

Calories	Protein	Sugar	Carbs

Saturday

Breakfast: ___________

Calories	Protein	Sugar	Carbs

Lunch: ___________

Calories	Protein	Sugar	Carbs

Dinner: ___________

Calories	Protein	Sugar	Carbs

Shopping List:

WEEKLY MEAL PLANNING

Month: __________________

Week: ① ② ③ ④

Sunday

Breakfast: __________________

Calories	Protein	Sugar	Carbs

Lunch: __________________

Calories	Protein	Sugar	Carbs

Dinner: __________________

Calories	Protein	Sugar	Carbs

Monday

Breakfast: __________________

Calories	Protein	Sugar	Carbs

Lunch: __________________

Calories	Protein	Sugar	Carbs

Dinner: __________________

Calories	Protein	Sugar	Carbs

Tuesday

Breakfast: __________________

Calories	Protein	Sugar	Carbs

Lunch: __________________

Calories	Protein	Sugar	Carbs

Dinner: __________________

Calories	Protein	Sugar	Carbs

Wednesday

Breakfast: __________________

Calories	Protein	Sugar	Carbs

Lunch: __________________

Calories	Protein	Sugar	Carbs

Dinner: __________________

Calories	Protein	Sugar	Carbs

Thursday

Breakfast: __________________

Calories	Protein	Sugar	Carbs

Lunch: __________________

Calories	Protein	Sugar	Carbs

Dinner: __________________

Calories	Protein	Sugar	Carbs

Friday

Breakfast: __________________

Calories	Protein	Sugar	Carbs

Lunch: __________________

Calories	Protein	Sugar	Carbs

Dinner: __________________

Calories	Protein	Sugar	Carbs

Saturday

Breakfast: __________________

Calories	Protein	Sugar	Carbs

Lunch: __________________

Calories	Protein	Sugar	Carbs

Dinner: __________________

Calories	Protein	Sugar	Carbs

Shopping List:

WEEKLY MEAL PLANNING

Month: _______________

Week:

(1) (2) (3) (4)

Sunday

Breakfast: _______________

Calories	Protein	Sugar	Carbs

Lunch: _______________

Calories	Protein	Sugar	Carbs

Dinner: _______________

Calories	Protein	Sugar	Carbs

Monday

Breakfast: _______________

Calories	Protein	Sugar	Carbs

Lunch: _______________

Calories	Protein	Sugar	Carbs

Dinner: _______________

Calories	Protein	Sugar	Carbs

Tuesday

Breakfast: _______________

Calories	Protein	Sugar	Carbs

Lunch: _______________

Calories	Protein	Sugar	Carbs

Dinner: _______________

Calories	Protein	Sugar	Carbs

Wednesday

Breakfast: _______________

Calories	Protein	Sugar	Carbs

Lunch: _______________

Calories	Protein	Sugar	Carbs

Dinner: _______________

Calories	Protein	Sugar	Carbs

Thursday

Breakfast: _______________

Calories	Protein	Sugar	Carbs

Lunch: _______________

Calories	Protein	Sugar	Carbs

Dinner: _______________

Calories	Protein	Sugar	Carbs

Friday

Breakfast: _______________

Calories	Protein	Sugar	Carbs

Lunch: _______________

Calories	Protein	Sugar	Carbs

Dinner: _______________

Calories	Protein	Sugar	Carbs

Saturday

Breakfast: _______________

Calories	Protein	Sugar	Carbs

Lunch: _______________

Calories	Protein	Sugar	Carbs

Dinner: _______________

Calories	Protein	Sugar	Carbs

Shopping List: